Weight Loss
Smart Workbook

How to lose weight by eating low carbs, calorie-controlled diet plan, exercises – walking, running, swimming, yoga & cycling

Table of Contents

Weight Loss Smart Workbook
How to lose weight by eating low carbs, calorie-controlled diet plan, exercises – walking, running, swimming, yoga & cycling

By M. A. Kabir

Copyright © 2015 by M. A. Kabir

Disclaimer

Who this book is for

I am predicting that you are interested in this book for one of the following reasons:

- You want to discover the tools and techniques of losing weight practically
- You want to lose weight because you are not happy with your current weight
- You want not to gain weight by knowing it in the first place
- You want to enhance your knowledge regarding not only losing weight but also controlling it
- You want to become practically successful in losing weight
- You want to help others to lose weight
- You are not looking for only motivations
- Others as well

Introduction

Greetings! Welcome to simple and straightforward but super practical ways of losing weight and controlling weight in your whole life. Right now, say hi to your excess body weight. Those extra weight is going to disappear in next few months. You have to struggle, work hard, be focused in doing so, but I strongly believe that you would successfully shed those unnecessary body weight.

Have you ever discovered that being heavy means carrying more than just the excess pounds?

When your weight is more than 250 pounds, you might feel that being heavy means carrying more than just the excess pounds. Weighing 350 plus pounds could be a barrier to having a positive career, get married, start a family, and move flexibly. Everywhere you might feel as well as realize unhappiness and discomfort because of being overweight. You must do something at your disposal to get rid of those pointless pounds in order to remain healthy and happy.

Even though a great number of reasons are there that transforms a person to become overweight. The key features can be:
- Less desire to control and limit eating habits
- Overeating by having snacks, fast food, beverages, sweets, chocolates, and so on
- Less attention to consumed meal, especially carbohydrate, beverages, and saturated fat
- Less awareness regarding weight gain, body fitness, and staying handsome or gorgeous
- Intake of calories is greater than expenditure of calories
- Less effective diet plan
- Lack of physical exercise
- Less interest and laziness to lose weight
- Hormones

You must do something consistently to stop following the above-mentioned patterns. Studies have verified that the well-organized approach to losing weight is calorie limitation, which means eating fewer calories.

Basal Metabolic Rate (BMR) + Thermic effect of food (TEF) + Physical Exercises = Total intake of calories (daily)

Did you ever calculate your daily calorie requirements?

For example, it can be around 2000 Calories or 2000 kcal daily. **Don't give up on awesome food and instead just try to decrease the quantity and frequency.** In that case, your total intake of calories can fluctuate between 1800 kcal and 2200 kcal.

There are a lot of overweight individuals, who passed their whole life, around the world without calculating their daily calorie requirements. A smart person should know how to control the balance with no trouble at all. However, that person must not miss calculating calories in a regular basis.

Always plan to burn off 200-300 kcal more than your total intake of calories for that day to lose weight. Try to burn off those 200-300 kcal more in doing physical exercises because your regular expenditure of calories through BMR and TEF would be automatic. So, your focus should be on eating low carbs, low fat excluding saturated fat as much as possible, following a calorie-controlled healthy diet plan, and physical exercises because a healthy diet should provide all your essential micronutrients.

Learning to control the intake of calories, nutrition, comfort eating, and regular physical exercise are key features. You won't change unless you decide to make your health as top priority.

Overweight causes illness

Sometimes we don't take proper actions to reduce weight. However, it is essential to keep losing weight in mind because being overweight can cause the following illness:

Coronary Heart Disease (CHD)

CHD is generally the result of a fat build-up within the wall surfaces in the coronary arteries throughout the heart.

The actual fat builds up inside the coronary arteries, known as atheroma, is consist of cholesterol and various waste materials. This fat build-up within the wall surfaces in the coronary arteries tends to make the blood vessels narrower, limiting the blood circulation towards the heart. This procedure is referred to as atherosclerosis and can be drastically elevated if someone:

- Have hypertension (high blood pressure)
- Have an increased blood cholesterol level

- Have diabetes
- Don't consider physical exercise
- Smoking
- Being overweight
- Having a family history of CHD

Fat produced by the liver, known as cholesterol, comes from the saturated fat in what we eat. Healthy and balanced cells require cholesterol; however, an excessive amount of cholesterol in the bloodstream can cause CHD. Cholesterol is transported inside the blood vessels by substances referred to as lipoproteins. Out of unique variations of lipoproteins, a couple of most important types are high-density lipoproteins (HDL) and low-density lipoproteins (LDL).

LDL carries cholesterol out of the liver and transports it to cells whereas HDL conveys cholesterol away from the cells and return it to the liver. LDL, known as bad cholesterol, is likely to build up within the wall surfaces in the coronary arteries, boosting your possibility of cardiovascular disease. HDL, known as good cholesterol, is broken down in the liver and delivered from the body as a waste material.

High Blood Pressure

Doctors and scientists are still researching to identify the actual cause of hypertension or high blood pressure. Several aspects that may increase your possibility of building primary hypertension:

- The possibility increases as you grow old
- Having a family history of high blood pressure
- Consuming a lot of alcohol
- A lot of smoking
- Overweight
- A higher quantity of food salt in regular meal and
- others

Insomnia

Sleeplessness or insomnia is often brought on by a variety of factors such as hypertension, base health issues, being overweight, drug, or alcohol use. Having a nap in the daytime, going to bed at different times, or without having rest before you go to sleep might give you trouble to have a sound sleep at night. Furthermore, an unhealthy surroundings might lead to insomnia, for example, an uncomfortable bed, or a bedroom which is very noisy, bright, warm or cold.

Stroke

Both strokes, ischemic strokes and hemorrhagic strokes, can have various reasons and impact the human brain in distinct behaviors. Ischemic strokes happen whenever a blood clot prevents blood circulation and oxygen to the brain. These kinds of blood clots generally form in places where the blood vessels happen to be narrowed or jammed as time passes by fat build up or plaques. On the other hand, hemorrhagic strokes happen whenever a blood vessel inside the head breaks and bleeds into the human brain. High blood pressure is identified as the primary reason of hemorrhagic strokes whereas the followings can cause ischemic strokes:

- high blood pressure
- high LDL cholesterol
- alcohol consumption
- diabetes and
- smoking

Are you overweight and focused to shed a significant amount of pounds by eating low-carbs, calorie-controlled diet plan, physical & cardio exercises such as walking, running, yoga, swimming, and cycling? Other physical, cardio and strength workout can be applied to lose weight as well. I hope that can be discussed in the next book.

Are you ready to carry on your top priority adventure to lose weight?

Let's start...

You have got the endless power, which is already existing in you, to change yourself. You definitely love yourself and want to see yourself beautiful, healthy and happy.

Action Plan

I want you to calculate and find out the following things right away if possible:

What is your total body weight just wearing underwear or bikini? Answer: ___ kg

If you measured your body weight as pounds then you can do the conversion given below.

1 pound / 1lb = 450 grams / 450 g

For example, if you weigh 200 pounds then your weight in kg would be
(200 x 450) / 1000 = 90 kg

What is your total body height? Answer: ___ cm

If you figured out your body height as inch then you can do the conversion given below.

1 inch = 2.5 centimeters / 2.5 cm

1 foot = 12 inches = 30 centimeters

For example, if your body height is 6 feet 2 inch then your height in cm would be
(6 x 30) + (2 x 2.5) = 185 cm

Wait! You need a log book right away. Please, prepare a fantastic log book to track your progress.

You are welcome to do the followings:

- Write down your current overall weight in the log book. If you don't know your exact weight right now then you need to measure your weight as soon as possible.
- Start your journey by writing down the current date and time.
- Are you following a diet plan? Write down the name of the diet plan and its starting time.
- Do you know how many calories you consume daily? Answer: circle → Yes / No
- Do you know how many calories you need to consume daily? Answer: circle → Yes/ No
- Are you performing activities such as walking, running, swimming, yoga, and cycling to lose weight? Write down the activity name, its total activity hours for a week, your own pros and cons for any of these activities such as "I am not comfortable with cycling and so on".

Chapter 01: Terms to calculate calories

Calories

What are Calories?
Are you fascinated to calculate or measure Calories? Why?

Because to lose weight, daily intake of calories should be less than daily burn off calories.

A calorie is a unit of energy which is used as a measurement for the amount of energy which food provides.

As stated by Google search, a calorie is a unit that is used to measure energy. The Calorie you see on a food package is actually a kilocalorie or **1,000 calories**. A Calorie (kcal) is the amount of energy needed to raise the temperature of 1 kilogram of water 1 degree Celsius.

According to the National Data Lab (NDL), most of the calorie values in the USDA and industry food tables are based on an indirect calorie estimation made using the so-called Atwater system. In this system, calories are not determined directly by burning the foods. Instead, the total caloric value is calculated by adding up the calories provided by the energy-containing nutrients: protein, carbohydrate, fat, and alcohol. Because carbohydrates contain some fiber that is not digested and utilized by the body, the fiber component is usually subtracted from the total carbohydrate before calculating the calories.

The following figures are used by the Atwater system, which were determined by burning and then averaging:

1 g of protein = 4 kcal
1 g of carbohydrate = 4 kcal
1 g of fat = 9 kcal
1 g of alcohol = 7 kcal

For example, if the label on a food packet shows that its nutrients are 10 g of carbohydrate (means 10 x 4 kcal = 50 kcal), 5 g of protein (means 5 x 4 kcal = 20 kcal), and 4.5 g of fat (means 4.5 x 9 kcal = 40.5 kcal) then the total amount of calories should be displayed as 100.5/100 kcal or 100.5/100 Calories approximately.

A complete discussion of this subject and the calories contained in foods may be found on the National Data Lab website at http://fnic.nal.usda.gov.

Occasionally fitness charts state that if you run for 1 kilometer then you will approximately burn 50 Calories. In fact, such 50 Calories is equal to 50x1000 = 50,000 calories or 50 kcal. The estimation of calories is provided within the package if it is a packaged food.

Calorie Counters

Is it an interesting term for you?
Do you want to find out how many calories you need to consume daily?
Are you curious to discover a calorie-controlled diet plan based on your calorie counter result? Why?

Because calorie-counting is the best way of losing weight.

I am guessing that most of us are already familiar with the term. To strengthen your own scientific research in relation to **daily intake of calories and burn off calories**, let yourself an opportunity to learn more about it just by browsing online when you might get some free time.

Action Plan

It is likely that you have access to a computer (desktop or laptop) or a mobile phone by which you are able to browse the internet, or you can visit a nearby cybercafé. You are welcome to do the followings (these steps are given by considering those people who didn't use online before):

- Open a browser such as Internet Explorer, Google Chrome, Mozilla Firefox, Opera, Safari, or etc.
- Type in your **browser's address bar** www.google.com and press enter
- When google search bar will show up, type in **calorie counters** within the search bar
- A list will come up in seconds related to your searched keywords.
- Visit a few top listed websites and fill up required fields to calculate your daily intake of calories

<u>**Note:**</u> Different websites calculate daily intake of calories by applying or taking various inputs from the user. After having results from at least five websites, you might have an idea of your required average daily intake of calories. An athlete in training needs a lot of calories compared to an average person and requirement of calories varies from person to persons

such as a vegetarian, pregnant woman, diabetic person, person on a low fat or low carbs diet. Look for the following features:

- BMR (Basal Metabolic Rate)
- Thermic effect of food
- Physical Activity

What is Basal Metabolic Rate (BMR)?

Basal metabolic rate (BMR) is the smallest rate of energy expenditure per unit time by endothermic animals at rest. The person should have the followings facts to measure BMR properly:

- In physically & psychologically undisturbed state
- In a thermally neutral environment (optional)
- In the post-absorptive state (i.e. not actively digesting food)

Factors:

- BMR decreases with age and with the decrease of lean body mass (LBM)

How to calculate BMR?

The Katch-McArdle Formula is used to calculate Resting Daily Energy Expenditure (RDEE):

$P = 370 + (21.6 \text{ x LBM})$

P = Total heat production at complete rest, kcal per day
LBM = Lean Body Mass in kg

For example:

If a 55-year-old woman weighing 130 pounds (59 kg), 5 feet 6 inches (168 cm) tall and has 30% body fat then her RDEE would be:

$P = 370 + (21.6 \text{ x LBM})$

Get rid of 30% body fat to calculate LBM
LBM = 59 − (59 x 30/100)
LBM = 59 -17.7
LBM = 41.3 kg

So, P = 370 + (21.6 x 41.3)
P = 1262.08

So, her RDEE = 1262.08 kcal per day

Using Katch-McArdle formula, without considering her body fat percentage BMR would be

LBM = (0.29569 x 59) + (0.41813 x 168) − 43.2933
LBM = 17.44571 + 70.24584 − 43.2933
LBM = 44.39825 kg

So, P = 370 + (21.6 x 44.39825)
P = 1329.0022

So, her RDEE = 1329 kcal per day

What is Body Mass Index (BMI)?

The Body Mass Index (BMI), defined as the body mass divided by the square of the body height, is the amount of tissue mass such as muscle, fat, and bone in a person. Normally, BMI value indicates whether an individual is underweight, normal, overweight or obese. A person's thickness or slimness can be mathematically measured by BMI.

BMI ranges:

Underweight is less than 18.5

Normal weight is 18.5 to 25

Overweight is 25 to 30

Obese is over 30

More detailed BMI and BMI Prime ranges:

Category	BMI range – kg/m²	BMI Prime
Very severely underweight	less than 15	less than 0.60
Severely underweight	from 15.0 to 16.0	from 0.60 to 0.64
Underweight	from 16.0 to 18.5	from 0.64 to

		0.74
Normal (healthy weight)	from 18.5 to 25	from 0.74 to 1.0
Overweight	from 25 to 30	from 1.0 to 1.2
Obese Class I (Moderately obese)	from 30 to 35	from 1.2 to 1.4
Obese Class II (Severely obese)	from 35 to 40	from 1.4 to 1.6
Obese Class III (Very severely obese)	over 40	over 1.6

Source: The table data is taken from Wikipedia.

Here, the standard value for BMI Prime, the ratio of body weight to the upper body weight limit, is 25. On the other hand, it has international variations.

For example, if someone calculates his or her BMI is equal to 30 then his or her BMI Prime would be 30/25 = 1.2 (Overweight)

How to calculate BMI?

BMI (m/f) = Body Weight (in kg) / (Height)^2 (in meter)

Or

BMI (m/f) = Body Weight (in pounds) / (Height)^2 (in inch)

What is Body Fat Percentage (BFP)?

The total mass of fat divided by total body mass is calculated as the body fat percentage (BFP) of a human or other living being. If metrics, for example, the waist circumference of a person is greater than 45% of their height then he or she might be included in the obese individuals. BFP openly computes a person's comparative body composition without regard to height or weight. To maintain an individual's life and reproductive system, essential body fat is indispensable.

Description	Women	Men
Essential fat	10–13%	2–5%
Athletes	14–20%	6–13%
Fitness	21–24%	14–17%
Average	25–31%	18–24%
Obese	32%+	25%+

How to calculate BFP?

Body fat % in Child = (1.51 x BMI) – (0.70 x Age) – (3.6 x sex) + 1.4

Body fat % in Adult = (1.20 x BMI) – (0.23 x Age) – (10.8 x sex) + 5.4

Here, for sex value:

Males = 1
Females = 0

For example, if a man, aged 32, calculates his BMI is equal to 30 (adult person) then his BFP would be:

His BFP = (1.20 x 30) – (0.23 x 32) – (10.8 x 1) + 5.4
His BFP = 36 – 7.36 – 10.8 + 5.4
His BFP = 23.24 % (average for men is 18-24%)

One thing to note down here is that even though that person is considered as overweight based on BMI table because his BMI is 30/25 = 1.2 (overweight) using BMI prime; however, he is found average (23.24%) from the BFP calculation. Therefore, it is better to use BFP instead of BMI to identify someone as an obese individual. In this case, he might be very muscular, lean (low body fat) individual who is being categorized as obese using BMI.

What is Lean Body Mass (LBM)?

Lean Body Mass is calculated by subtracting body fat weight from total body weight, a component of body composition. The formula:

LBM = Body Weight – Body Fat

How to calculate LBM?

LBM (male) = [0.32810 x Body Weight (kilograms)] + [0.33929 x Body Height (cm)] – 29.5336

LBM (female) = [0.29569 x Body Weight (kilograms)] + [0.41813 x Body Height (cm)] – 43.2933

What is Thermic effect of food (TEF)?

Thermic effect of food (TEF), also described as the energy used in the distribution of nutrients and metabolic processes in the liver, is the amount of energy expenditure above the resting metabolic rate (RMR) due to the cost of processing food for use and storage. Approximately 50% energy from glucose breakdown is instantaneously transformed to heat.

Factors:

- The thermic effect of food is raised to 7-8 Calories / 7-8 kcal per hour by both aerobic training and anaerobic weight training.
- TEF is little to no effect on meal frequency.
- For the majority of people, Thermic effect of food (TEF) lasts greater than 6 hours according to the American Journal of Clinical Nutrition.

How to calculate TEF?

In general, 10% of the total daily intake of calories can be measured as TEF. It should be noted that protein is hard to process compared to dietary fat. For this reason, protein has much larger thermic effect whereas dietary fat has a very little thermic effect.

So, if your total daily intake of calories is equal to 2000 Calories or 2000 kcal then your TEF would be around 200 Calories or 200 kcal.

What is Physical Activity Level (PAL)?

By dividing someone's, excluding pregnant women and lactating adult, Total Energy Expenditure (TEE), which is based on his or her BMR, TEF and physical exercises including all other daily physical activities, in an entire day by his or her that day's Basal Metabolic Rate (BMR), the Physical Activity Level (PAL) can be mathematically measured.

Lifestyle	Example	PAL
Extremely inactive	Cerebral Palsy patient	<1.40
Sedentary	Office worker getting little or no exercise	1.40-1.69
Moderately active	Construction worker or the person running one hour daily	1.70-1.99
Vigorously active	Agricultural worker (non-mechanized) or a person swimming two hours daily	2.00-2.40
Extremely active	Competitive cyclist	>2.40

Source: The table data is taken from Wikipedia

How to calculate PAL?

PAL = TEE (based on 24 hours) / BMR

For example, if someone's BMR, total intake of calories and total energy expenditure are 1500 Calories or 1500 kcal, 1800 kcal on Sunday, and 2200 kcal on Sunday (BMR-1500 kcal + TEF-150 kcal + Physical Exercises including all other activities-550 kcal) respectively, then his or her PAL would be:

PAL = 2200 kcal / 1500 kcal
PAL = 1.467 (approx.) (Sedentary active)

Chapter 02: Calorie-controlled Diet Plan

You might eat less food, or only particular types of food because you want to become thinner. This plan can be expressed as a diet plan when you have an existing realistic goal like losing 5% of your body fat in 6 weeks.

Diets can differ sometimes such as balanced diet (a combination of the correct types and amounts of food), crash diet (a way of losing body weight quickly by eating very little), or starvation diet (a way of eating only a very small amount of food in order to lose weight quickly).

What is a calorie-controlled diet plan?

A calorie-controlled diet plan means the total intake of calories is specifically controlled by you based on your daily expenditure of calories. In this diet plan, you will take 200-300 less kcal each day to make it a steady healthy calorie-controlled diet to lose weight. Here, you must calculate your daily intake of calories and burns off calories.

For example: On Saturday you figured that you'd do certain activities and at the end of that day your total caloric expenditure would be 2200 Calories / 2200 kcal based on your BMR (including BFP), TEF and Physical Exercises. So, you'd eat between 1900 kcal and 2000 kcal on Saturday. On Sunday, it can be different based on your caloric expenditure.

To become successful in this plan, you should maintain the simple formula:

Daily intake of calories <= Daily burns off calories

Why had a calorie-controlled diet plan?

You'd automatically lose weight if you are strictly following a healthy diet, which takes care of all essential nutrients, without a lot of physical exercises. However, to lose weight much more efficiently, a superior approach is combining such diet into calorie-controlled diet plan including varieties of physical exercises.

It is based on scientific, mathematical and medical considerations. All you have to do is to make sure you are following a balanced, healthy and suitable diet plan that covers all important mini-micro nutrients.

Action Plan

Let's find out how many calories you need to consume daily...

For this you need to know three things:

- Body Weight (in kg): _____ kg
- Body Height (in cm): _____ cm
- Body Fat Percentage (in kg): _____ kg

Afterward, you need to do addition on followings:

- BMR (considering BFP)
- TEF (10% of total intake of calories)
- Physical Exercises

To calculate BFP, you need to know BMI

For example: If your body weight is 200 pounds and body height is 6 feet 2 inch then your BMI would be

BW = 200 pounds or 90 kg
BH = 6 feet 2 inch or 185 cm = 1.85 m

BMI = BW (in kg) / (BH)^2 (in meter)
BMI = 90 / (1.85)^2 = 90 / 3.4225 = 26.297 (based on BMI chart it is overweight)

Now, you can calculate your BFP, guessing age = 30, sex = male

Age = 30
Sex = male = 1 (for female it should be 0)

BFP (adult) = (1.20 x BMI) − (0.23 x Age) − (10.8 x sex) + 5.4
BFP = (1.20 x 26.297) − (0.23 x 30) − (10.8 x 1) + 5.4
BFP = 31.5564 − 6.9 − 10.8 + 5.4
BFP = 36.9564 − 17.7
BFP = 19.2564 or body fat = 19.2564 %

Now, you can calculate BMR (including BFP)

P = 370 + (21.6 x LBM)

Where, LBM = Body Weight − Body Fat

So, P = 370 + [21.6 x {90 − (90 x 19.2564 / 100}]

Because, Body Fat is 19.2565 % of Body Weight

P = 370 + [21.6 x {90 − 17.33}]
P = 370 + [21.6 x 72.67]
P = 370 + 1569.672
P = 1939.672 kcal

So, your BMR is 1939.67 kcal and if you are doing very little physical exercises where it requires only 200 kcal then

Your BMR + Physical Exercise = 1939.67 kcal + 200 kcal = 2139.67 kcal (without TEF)

Including TEF, (by guessing that your total intake of calories is 2000 kcal)
So TEF should be = 10 % of 1939.67 kcal = 190 kcal (approximately)

In the above mentioned example, the character (Sex = male, Age = 30, BW = 90 kg, BH = 185cm), who burns off 200 kcal by doing physical exercise on Saturday, need to consume the following amount of calories on Saturday:

Total intake of calories (on Saturday) = BMR + TEF + Physical Exercise
= 1939.67 kcal + 190 kcal (10 % of 1939.67) + 200 kcal (physical exercises done on Saturday)
= 2329.67 kcal

Based on the calculation the character needs to consume 2330 kcal on Saturday. You must be clear that it is not his daily calorie requirement. Your calorie requirement differs on daily physical exercise or physical labor.

Suppose, the character burned off 500 kcal on Sunday by doing only physical exercises such as running, walking, yoga, swimming and bicycling then his total intake of calories on Sunday would be
= 1939.67 kcal + 190 kcal (10 % of 1939.67) + 500 kcal (physical exercises done on Sunday)
= 2629.67 kcal

In a calorie-controlled diet plan, you should take 200-300 less kcal each day (by calculating that day's total intake of calories) to make it a steady healthy calorie-controlled diet to lose weight.

How are you going to control your daily intake of calories?

To control daily intake of calories, you need to have a better understanding regarding how much work you are going to do on a weekday and how many calories you require to do so. If you can manage to calculate your total daily energy expenditure (BMR +TEF + Physical Exercise + All Other Activities) and calories in everyday meals then you would be able to control your daily intake of calories not only to lose weight but also to balance it in your entire life.

All other activities besides physical exercise are very important that includes your work related and normal regular life activities. Energy expenditure in all other activities is a huge area to cover. But it is definitely short for you because you are not involved in all those activities. So, you need to figure out how many calories you are burning by doing your regular work related activities excluding physical exercises. After studying this book, I'm hoping that you would understand how to control your daily intake of calories.

How are you going to calculate calories in everyday meals?

Calculating calories in everyday meals is the hardest part because most of the time we don't have the opportunity when we consume food or drink from outside, and time for calculation at all. In the beginning, it would seem to be very complex and boring. But if you do this for at least one or two weeks then you would surely be able to do it much more quickly afterward. You need to know or have three things:

1. How many calories are there in per gram food type?
2. List of food showing calories per 100 gram
3. Small electronic machine to calculate food weight

You already know the first part:
1 g of protein = 4 kcal
1 g of carbohydrate = 4 kcal
1 g of fat = 9 kcal
1 g of alcohol = 7 kcal

You can get a lot of charts, tables, or an illustrating list of food along with calories per 100 gram, from online. These files are in pdf or spreadsheet format and free to download. A lot of websites are there to help you calculate calories as well. Most of the packaged food contains a list of caloric details. You can purchase one small electronic machine to calculate food weight manually at home. If you do take some food and drink from outside in a regular basis then you need to calculate those calories only one time. In time, you will have a better approach to do it more easily and quickly.

Chapter 03: Eating Low Carbs

A good diet plan should have all available micronutrients in order to replenish our daily requirements without adding extra pounds.

Low Carbs Intakes

It is really essential for us to take enough carbs (from 50 to 100 grams, provides 200 to 400 kcal) in a regular basis as we get our regular energy from carbohydrates. In addition, carbs generate thyroid hormone production which is essential to balance maintaining our metabolic process and fat burning process. However, an excess amount of carbs intake does directly increase extra pounds in the form of fat.

On the other hand, very low carbs intakes can have negative impact such as

- It drains glycogen levels in your body. As a result, you might experience very low energy to perform daily activities and your muscles are less healthy, firm or toned.
- It reduces the production of thyroid hormone. In doing so, our body metabolism, the fat burning process will be decreased.
- It can increase cortisol hormone level which usually creates an environment to store body weight including water weight and burn up muscle tissues to regulate the required energy.

Low Fat Intakes

No matter what diet plan we follow, we are constantly consuming fat. Fat intakes can be of different types such as saturated fats, monounsaturated fats, polyunsaturated fats, and trans fats. Out of these fats, not all fats are bad for our health.

A great number of organizations including American Heart Association recommend that saturated fat intake should be less than 7% of daily intake of calories. Intake of saturated fats increase the chances of cardiovascular health diseases whereas polyunsaturated fats decrease it. Monounsaturated fats help to reduce LDL cholesterol, anger, heart diseases, stroke, and irritability. Polyunsaturated fats consist of omega-3 and omega-6 fatty acids which are effective to reduce heart diseases and to accelerate muscle tissue recovery. Trans fats are generally produced industrially by the partial hydrogenation of vegetable fats in order to preserve the taste and quality of food such as snack food, packaged baked goods, cookies, and fried food. Researches done by various organizations show that trans fats are not good for health at all, not essential and it directly increases LDL cholesterol and coronary heart diseases.

Fruits, whole grains, vegetables, poultry, fish, low-fat dairy products can easily replace the required nutrients instead of saturated fats, sugary foods, and beverages. Therefore, it is considered wise to reduce the number of saturated fats and trans fats from your diet plan. The following list might give you a head start:

Food	Saturated	Mono-unsaturated	Poly-unsaturated
	As weight percent (%) of total fat		
Cooking oils			
Canola oil	8	64	28
Corn oil	13	24	59
Olive oil	7	78	15
Sunflower oil	11	20	69
Soybean oil	15	24	58
Peanut oil	17	46	32
Rice bran oil	25	38	37
Coconut oil	87	13	1
Dairy products			
Cheese, regular	64	29	3
Cheese, light	60	30	0
Milk, whole	62	28	4
Milk, 2%	62	30	0
Ice cream, gourmet	62	29	4
Ice cream, light	62	29	4
Meats			
Beef	33	38	5
Ground sirloin	38	44	4
Pork chop	35	44	8
Ham	35	49	16
Chicken breast	29	34	21
Chicken	34	23	30
Turkey breast	30	20	30
Turkey drumstick	32	22	30
Fish, orange roughly	23	15	46
Salmon	28	33	28
Hot dog, beef	42	48	5
Hot dog, turkey	28	40	22

Burger, fast food	36	44	6
Cheeseburger, fast food	43	40	7
Breaded chicken sandwich	20	39	32
Grilled chicken sandwich	26	42	20
Sausage, Polish	37	46	11
Sausage, turkey	28	40	22
Pizza, sausage	41	32	20
Pizza, cheese	60	28	5
Nuts			
Almonds dry roasted	9	65	21
Cashews dry roasted	20	59	17
Macadamia dry roasted	15	79	2
Peanut dry roasted	14	50	31
Pecans dry roasted	8	62	25
Flaxseeds, ground	8	23	65
Sesame seeds	14	38	44
Soybeans	14	22	57
Sunflower seeds	11	19	66
Walnuts dry roasted	9	23	63
Sweets and baked goods			
Candy, chocolate bar	59	33	3
Candy, fruit chews	14	44	38
Cookie, oatmeal raisin	22	47	27
Cookie, chocolate chip	35	42	18
Cake, yellow	60	25	10
Pastry, Danish	50	31	14
Fats added during cooking or at the table			
Butter, stick	63	29	3
Butter, whipped	62	29	4
Margarine, stick	18	39	39
Margarine, tub	16	33	49
Margarine, light tub	19	46	33
Lard	39	45	11
Shortening	25	45	26
Chicken fat	30	45	21
Beef fat	41	43	3
Dressing, blue cheese	16	54	25
Dressing, light	14	24	58

Italian			
Other			
Egg yolk fat	36	44	16
Avocado	16	71	13

Source: The above list is taken from Wikipedia.

Action Plan

Don't think that it very hard or impossible to lose weight if you follow a good diet plan and do exercise in a regular basis. Calculate you daily intake of calories. Track down everything you eat and drink.

Your present situation can be of two types:
1) You do need to lose weight because you have extra weight
2) You are in a fantastic shape and you don't want to gain weight

To lose weight:

Daily total intake of calories < Daily total energy expenditure (BMR + TEF + Physical Exercise + All other activities)

To control present fitness:

Daily total intake of calories <= Daily total energy expenditure (BMR + TEF + Physical Exercise + All other activities)

Chapter 04: Walking to lose weight

Walking is a fantastic way to lose weight for people who are more than 350 pounds because they might be uncomfortable with running, swimming, cycling and physical exercises including other cardio exercises. To dispose of a considerable quantity of fat, walking is truly a long method that involves about 3-6 months depending on your targeted amount of weight. If you are determined to lose 20 lbs or 9 kg excess weight just by walking then, it is possible to do so within 6-9 months period combining speed walking, willpower, and tenacity. It really depends on regular walking and with a standard pace. Walking 3 miles in an hour (at 3 miles/hour or 4.8 km/hour) each day, 6 times in each week, can help decrease excess weight by roughly 0.45 kg or 1 pound every week. It may vary based on your overall existing body weight. Therefore, you need to keep track of your body weight and the change you made within a week.

You are able to utilize going for walks, not merely for any practical reason to travel, but instead for enjoyment and enhanced well-being by including walking straight into your everyday schedule. Walking is a type of aerobic fitness exercise where aerobic stands for those exercises that are performed at a contented speed to make sure that the muscles have adequately accessible oxygen. In case you are gasping for air, you are performing anaerobic fitness exercise. Go walking at a speed rate which is quick; however, it would not stop you from speaking to a co-walker in a usual way.

Health Benefits of Walking

Systematic and consistent walking provides an immediate influence on the muscle flexibility and cardiovascular system by

- Minimizing the chance of heart disease and stroke
- Decreasing hypertension (high blood pressure)
- Lowering LDL cholesterol levels in bloodstream
- Escalating bone structure thickness, therefore protecting against osteoporosis and unwanted side effects of osteoarthritis
- getting rid of back problems

Taking walks in a regular basis can enhance your overall well-being and durability. Based on the US survey, the standard of lifestyle increases significantly besides longevity just by regular walking.

Action Plan

Please, check your medical background and current medication before attempting to go for an intensive cardio exercise namely walking, running and cycling to lose weight. In addition, consult with your doctor to make sure you are fully fit for your desired duration of walking if you have high blood pressure, pregnancy, physical injury in specific areas, and etc.

According to estimates, if your weight is 200 pounds and you continue walking for an hour at 3 miles/hour or 4.8 km/hour then you will approximately burn 250-300 kcal (1050 – 1260 kilojoules) including BMR. A scientific study revealed that short walkers, who are splitting their walking hours, are getting better result compared to long walkers. So, it should be better to walk early in the morning for half an hour and then in the evening for half an hour again instead of walking for an hour in the morning.

If you are desperate and want to shed 1 pound in a week just by walking and nothing else then you should do the followings:

1) To burn 3500-3600 kcal just by walking you need to walk for approximately 12-15 hours at 3 miles/hour or 4.8 km/hour in a week. So, you can do it either by walking for 2 hours daily in 7 days or 3 hours in 5 days. Find your available free time and do your unique adjustments.
2) Calculate your daily intake of calories (BMR + TEF + Physical Exercises) and make sure to burn 500-600 kcal more daily by walking. Please, see the topics from where you can calculate your BMR and TEF.
3) Have your breakfast and set off for walking. Split your walking hours twice in each day instead of walking for 2 hours intensively. Carry a bottle of water to keep yourself hydrated. Wear light clothes and a comfortable pair of walking shoes. Pick up a wonderful area where you will enjoy fresh air and environment.
4) Get a friend or partner to stay out of boredom and loneliness. Use electronic devices to listen to the news, radio stations, sports, music, audio books, or work related audio materials.

Obviously wise approach is to combine other physical exercises besides walking to stay out of boredom and to implement it in your current lifestyle permanently.

You are not eating the same quantity of food every day, so calculate your intake of calories for that particular day and increase or decrease your time for walking. Mix and match with other activities such as running, swimming, yoga, cycling, and heavy cardio exercises if necessary to lose weight at a significant rate. Try to avoid unnecessary injury or pain by not going for intensive walking. The treadmill can be used to do it indoors.

To note down your regular progress, you are welcome to create your own weekly chart of walking schedule besides other physical exercises.

Chapter 05: Running to lose weight

Running is a first-rate way to burn off excess calories. It is a serious physical exercise; stamina varies from person to person. Any person might announce, he or she wish to slim down by running. However, numerous exact same individuals who say that wind up less committed, determined, and postpone their activity concerning running to lose weight.

Running to get rid of a substantial quantity of weight is actually a lengthy procedure that includes about 3-4 months. However, it is a much faster and effective way to shed pounds compared to walking and yoga. So, if you decide to drop extra pounds quickly then I would suggest you give more time here.

Health Benefits of Running

Running on a regular basis just for a couple of minutes can provide the following magical benefits:

- Increases longevity by around three years which is scientifically proven
- Boosts stamina, muscle strength and flexibility, body metabolism and fitness
- Minimizing the chance of heart disease and stroke
- Decreases hypertension (high blood pressure), insomnia or sleeplessness
- Heightens mood, brain activity and performance, self-healing heart

Action Plan

According to general estimates, if your weight is 200 pounds and you continue running for an hour at 6 miles/hour or 9.6 km/hour then you will approximately burn 500-600 kcal including BMR.

Did you check your medical background and current medication to justify you're good to carry on desired running schedules or medically fit?
(For example: If you continue running for about 1 hour at 6-10 miles/hour or 9.6-16 km/hour then you will be perfectly fit without any sort of problem or injury)

It will be wise to purchase a comfortable pair of running shoes, which might take $50-$100 from the very beginning to minimize injury and cheer yourself up. If your budget is to minimize expenses then you can pick parks and trails instead of a comfortable gym. Your primary objective should be eating fresh food and vegetables, running on a regular basis, increasing stamina, creating an effective running schedule and sticking to it in order to lose the noteworthy amount of excess body weight.

What is your desired amount of calories to burn by running based on your daily calorie intakes? Answer: __ kcal
(For example Saturday 500 kcal, Sunday 600 kcal, Monday 400 kcal because your daily intake of calories changes)

Actually you can just eat 200 – 300 fewer calories per day to reduce the amount of burn off calories by running or other physical exercises.

How much weight would you like to lose by running? Answer: ____ pounds
(For example 50 lbs or 22.5 kg)

Your estimation should be like 50 lbs to lose in 2-3 months. Please, increase your duration of running and speed very slowly based on your stamina and don't go for unorthodox running because you will feel terrible and you should not lose a lot of weight in a short period of time.

Don't forget to use your log book wisely to track down all your progress.

How to start running as a beginner?

You can do the followings to give yourself a head start:

- You need to have a clear mindset regarding how many pounds you want to lose.
- Don't attempt to run for a long time in the beginning and instead increase duration and distance slowly based on your endurance.
- Create a habit of walking on a regular basis to warm yourself up, afterward prepare for jogging & running.
- You can start running in a gymnasium, fitness center, an open environment where you would enjoy great scenery, perhaps in nearby parks or local trails, and fresh air, according to your comfort zones.
- Create a habit of eating healthy food such as fresh fruits, low carbs, low fats, food with low glycemic index and vegetables instead of the high amount of carbohydrate, saturated and trans fats, snacks, chocolates, junk food, beverages, or processed food because you will need fuel for running.

- Don't force yourself to go for extra mileage, when running would come to an end for that day unless you're absolutely sure that you will stay fit without avoiding injury.
- You need to give attention to stay away from the side effects of running.

Optional tips

You can ask one of your family members, friends, neighbors, or find one who is also willing to lose weight and stay fit by running so that both of you can do the running altogether to have a great time instead of running lonely.

You can use your Walkman, keep the volume down and listen to your favorite things such as radio stations, news, music, and work related things.

Use the combination of multiple great locations or routes, a fantastic comfortable pair of running shoes, jogging or light dress, fresh air to inhale and exhale, excellent time for running (early in the morning would be the best choice if you are not somehow busy every day in a week), regular exercises to increase stamina gradually.

Advanced Stage Techniques

To overcome running to lose weight common mistakes:

- Eat before running:
  - Eat your breakfast before running and carry a bottle of water to keep you hydrated because exercise is supposed to speed up your metabolism and you will need the required energy.

- Change workout:
  - If you feel it is easy for you to run for half an hour at 6 miles/hour, your running workout should be changed from time to time. In this case, you will not burn off calories as expected because your body metabolism will be adjusted. So, increase time and speed slowly to add up a bit more.

- Go faster instead of longer:
  - Always try to increase the intensity of a workout, cardio or other, instead of going for a long duration. So if you are planning to run for 1 hour at 6 miles/hour pace when your

stamina supports you then try to increase the pace like 8-10 miles/ hour and run for 30-45 minutes. You can try it in a treadmill or elliptical machine as well.

- Mix other cardio:
  - You will have a much better and faster result if you can add weight lifting & sprinting for a short period of time, cycling at a high intensity and others in the gym. These will impact on your metabolism in mini-micro areas which helps to burn more calories and proper muscle growth. Your entire body must rejuvenate required ATP (energy), transform lactic acid which is created throughout workout straight into glucose, and recover your blood hormonal imbalance right after powerful exercises.

- Don't run too much:
  - Medically, a hormone named cortisol is released when you perform workouts. Among all cortisol, prolonged stress and chronic cortisol may result in insulin resistance that makes you preserve abdominal fat in contradiction of your running to lose weight or scheduled plan. So, stay consistent about running based on your desired calories to burn.

- Take running injuries seriously:
  - You must watch out for any side effects of running and injury with proper care.

Side effects of running

- Black toenails:
  - Bleeding underneath the toenails while running may arise this problem. This happens because of ill-fitting shoe or too-small footwear. A comfortable well-filled pair of running shoes or a size larger might be the solution.

- Cackling knees:
  - Cackling knees, causes pain around or just behind the kneecaps, is actually patellofemoral pain syndrome. Sitting with bent knees, squatting, running, climbing, or descending stairs for a long time can evolve this suffering. You can do additional exercises, for example, straight leg raises and stretches in order to restore your knee.

- Dead butt syndrome:
    - Dead butt syndrome, affects distance runners and is formerly known as gluteus medius tendinosis. This typically starts off within the glutes and travels through the rear of the leg, therefore it may intensify as time passes in case you deal with it as necessary. You need to consult with your doctor to follow-up the appropriate treatment.

- Runner's face:
    - Runner's face usually impacts people aged over 40 who lose a lot of fatty tissue underneath their facial skin. It may cause accelerated development of skin laxity and deepen of wrinkles.

- Self-healing heart:
    - After an endurance running incident, the heart of a runner might be enlarged and the functions of the right ventricle can be reduced. According to scientists, running is healthy and the functions of the right ventricle will be healed automatically within a week.

Chapter 06: Yoga to lose weight

To perform the following yoga poses comfortably, you need a **soft yoga mat** or **carpeted space**.

Health Benefits of Yoga

Different types of yoga poses create effects on various parts of the human body such as feet, knees, thighs, abs, torso, shoulders, back, arms, palms, neck, and head. Yoga poses are comparatively slow in relation to weight loss, but effective in following ways:

- Strengthens muscle and its flexibility
- Tones or shapes various sections of human body
- Helps to learn how to channel and control flow of energy
- Some decrease hypertension (high blood pressure), stress, anxiety
- Increases stamina, self-control, meditation, physical immunity, body metabolism and fitness
- Less injurious, easy to perform
- Intensifies sexual performance, healing power

Yoga practitioners can experience other benefits besides the above-mentioned benefits as well.

Hover Pose (Push-up)

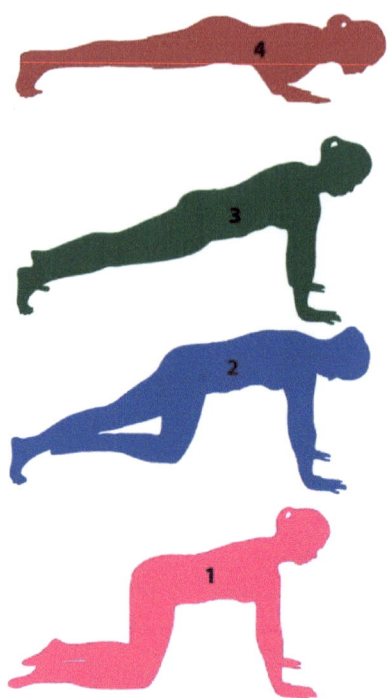

Avoid: You would be well-advised to stay away from this particular pose if you have any sort of arms or shoulder injury.

In step 1-3, this pose is actually the push-up (a physical exercise in which you lie flat with your face towards the floor and try to push up your body with your arms while keeping your legs and your back straight) exercise. Follow the above-mentioned image, position on hand & toes together with arms straight, hands underneath shoulders, and the entire body in a straight line.

Step 4 - During breathe out, lower your entire body in straight line and move downwards, keeping arms & elbows near your body, and instead of touching the floor maintains a little gap. You can hold your hover posture for 3-10 seconds each time before returning from step 4 to step 3.

Repeat: 5-15 times, hold your hover posture for 3-10 seconds each time

Benefits: This is a popular exercise to strengthen your arms, shoulders, and back.

Chair Pose (Utkatasana)

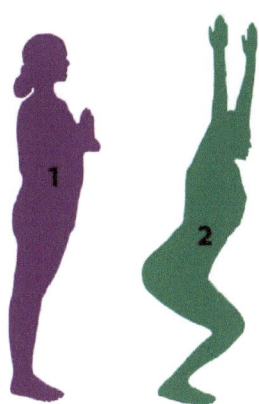

Avoid: You would be well-advised to stay away from this particular pose if you have any sort of knee or back injury.

In step 1-2, stand up on the ground, keep your back straight, your feet alongside one another with no gaps (see the above-mentioned image), breathe in slowly and lift your both hands above your head towards the ceiling, palms are pointed to one another, breathe out slowly and settle-back around forty-five degrees angle, bend your torso, maintain knees right behind toes (in the beginning keep knees in front of toes) and abdominal muscles constricted to aid your back, look ahead of you. You can hold this posture for a few breaths if possible and afterward get back to step 1 when you're done.

Repeat: 10-15 times, hold your chair posture for 15-30 seconds each time

Benefits: This exercise might help to firm up your legs, upper thighs, arms, and buttocks.

Tree Pose (Vrksasana)

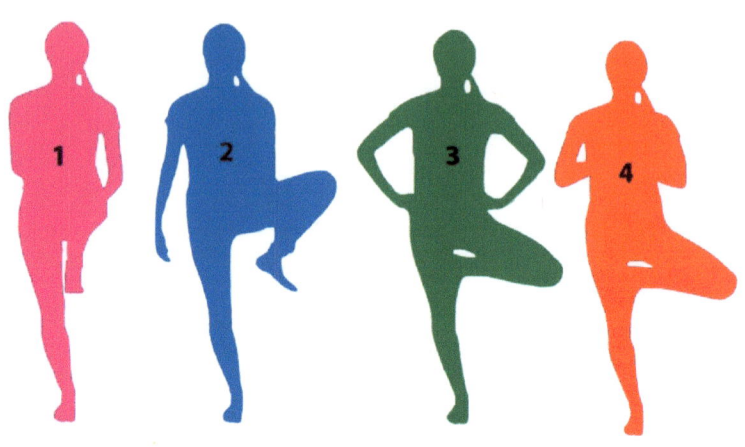

Avoid: You would be well-advised to stay away from this particular pose if you have any sort of knee or leg injury.

Step 1 - Tree pose is pretty simple standing pose. Transfer your entire body weight onto one leg and lift your other knee by lifting it close to your chest (step 1). Try to balance and hold this posture for a few seconds.

Step 2 - Now turn your lifted leg out from your hips (just like step 2 within the picture) and bring your foot to the inner thigh on your standing leg. Remember to place it onto your shin if your lifted foot does not get to your inner thigh (close to pelvis) and not to place it on the knee of your standing leg. Try to maintain the toes of your standing leg forward and press the foot of your lifted leg into your inner thigh as well as press your inner thigh into the sole of your lifted foot.

In step 3, you can move both hands on your hips and balance your position nicely without taking help by using a chair or wall.

Step 4 - From here you can do either bring your hands to meet in front of the heart center or slowly raise your hands above your head. You can focus on one single spot in front of you, hold this posture for about 1 minute each time, and take a few breaths steadily. Be sure you are standing straightly and keep the energy flowing upwards. When you are done, release your lifted foot and set it down on the ground. Move your legs for a few while to relax.

Benefits: This exercise strengthens the muscles in your standing leg, specifically your upper thighs, ankles, and kneecaps. It can help to enhance your feeling and sense of balance.

Plank Pose (Kumbhakasana)

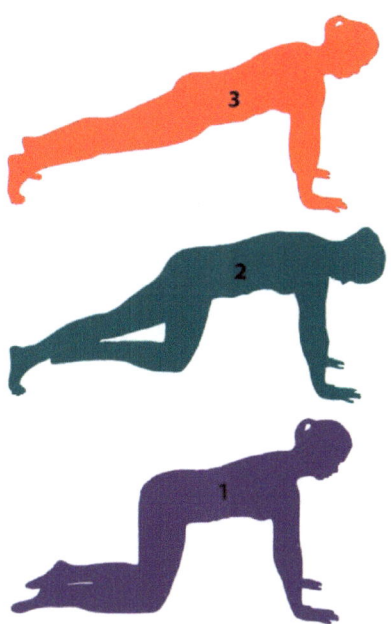

Avoid: You would be well-advised to stay away from this particular pose if you have any sort of arms or shoulder injury.

This pose is similar like hover exercise. Follow the above-mentioned image (step 1-2), position on hand & toes together with arms straight, hands underneath shoulders, and the entire body in a straight line (step 3). You can hold your plank posture as long as you want before returning from step 3 to step 1. To create variations, you can try to lift one of your legs upwards. Take extra care when you are going after variations to give yourself a bit of challenge, please.

Repeat: 5-15 times, hold your plank posture for 30-60 seconds each time

Benefits: This is a popular exercise to strengthen your toes, arms, shoulders, and back.

Side Plank Pose (Vasishtasana)

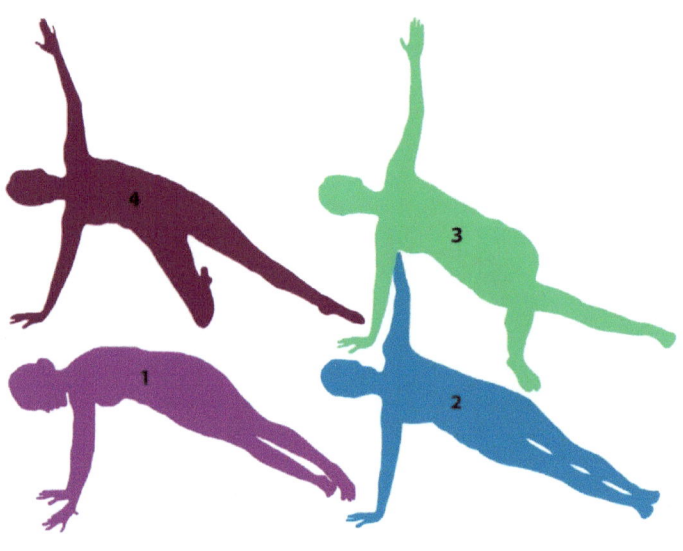

Avoid: You would be well-advised to stay away from this particular pose if you have arms, legs, and shoulder injuries or hypertension.

Get started by going for push-up and slowly come into plank posture (see plank pose) where two big toes have to be together side by side and spike the heels towards the back. Check to see that your body is in the same alignment along with your hips and pelvis.

In step 1, lift your right palm and place it on the center line of the ground slightly ahead from your shoulder point. Now press your body weight on the right palm and turn your left foot onto the right outer edge of your foot and stack it on your right foot.

In step 2, Keep balancing your position on your right palm, inhale and slowly lift your left hand towards the ceiling by moving the energy to flow from your right hand to left hand. Try not to let your hips and pelvis down and to keep your head straight together with your spine and find stability on your right shoulder. Hold your posture for about 30-45 seconds, exhale and put your left palm down on the ground and balance on your both hands. A bit harder technique can be slowly lifting your left leg as up as possible just after raising your left hand.

Step 3 - Another variation can be done instead of gently lifting your left hand. Just after balancing on your right palm, lift your left knee from the stacked position and place the sole of the left foot in front of your hips. Here your hips and pelvis will go down; however, raise them upward and try to position as best as you can. Now inhale, slowly lift your left hand and raise it all the way up or place it on your left waist.

Step 4 - Another variation can be done by bending your knees down on the ground from the push-up position. From here you can start swinging the right toe towards the right side of the ground. Maintain your left leg straight just like stacking your foot in the very first side plank pose. Start pressing on the right knee, keep balancing on your right palm and continue trying to raise your left hand towards the ceiling.

Benefits: This pose is a full value strengthener because you are going to get full body experience by performing it. It is great to assess your yoga practice as a beginner. It is not only for wrist and arms strength but also for getting the pelvis in line and finding integrity in the body.

Half-moon Pose (Ardha Chandraasana)

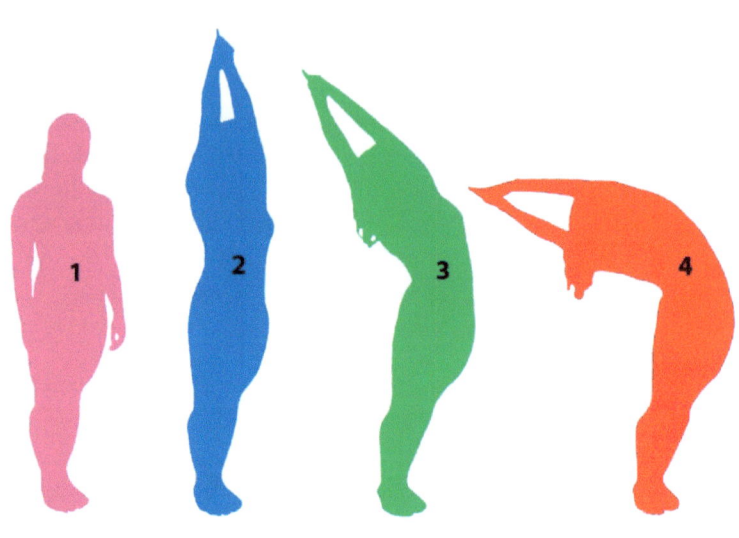

Avoid: You would be well-advised to stay away from this particular pose if you have any sort of backbone injury, stomach illness, or hypertension.

Step 1 - Start with your toes and knees together by squeezing your feet together.

Step 2 - Now lift your arms over your head towards the ceiling, touch your index fingers and keep it out while thumbs are crossed.

In step 3, push your hips forward and lean your torso back by stretching your spine with your own muscle. Get a deep breath and bend your body to the right side and push your hips beyond your flexibility if possible.

In step 4, hold your half-moon posture for a little while like 10-15 seconds and return to your standing position by keeping the arms raised and continue breathing before trying it again to the left side.

Benefits: This exercise might help you firm up legs, upper & inner thighs, abs, and buttocks. Added stretch might shape and tone your abdominal muscles. It can be done early in the morning to help warm up your spine.

Bridge Pose (Setubandhasana)

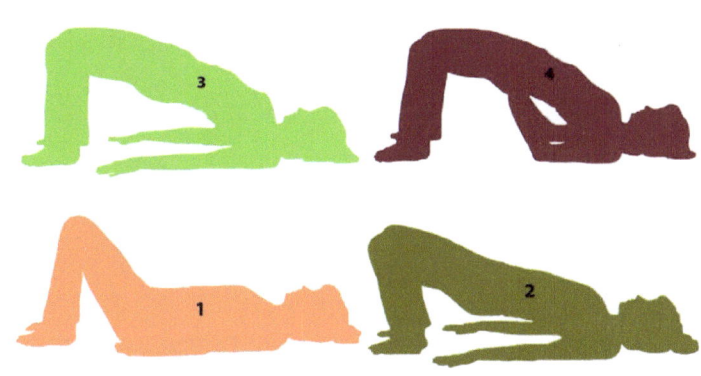

Avoid: You would be well-advised to stay away from this particular pose if you have any sort of neck, chest, and back injury.

Step 1 - Get started by lying down on the back together with your legs flat on the ground. Now bring your feet parallel to each other and pull them close to your hips to enable you to touch the heels using your own fingers. Don't worry if you can't bring your feet near your hips. Maintain your hands alongside your body together with palms down. You need to press your upper arms and shoulder down as flat on the ground.

In step 2-3, breathe out, start lifting your chest bone upward slowly along with your hips and create an arch. Continue to keep your head and neck fixed on the ground and don't attempt to move your posture on the left, right, feet direction or head direction while you're controlling your lifted position. Hold on to this posture for about one minute and have a few breaths.

Step 4 - You can interlace your fingers behind your back on the ground as well. If possible press the forearms down on the ground in order to lift the chest more. Another idea is to position your fingers directly below your hips to support your lifted position. When you are done, you may move your hips down on the ground and create gaps between your feet to relax a bit more and enable your entire body to get its balance again.

Benefits: This exercise can help to change mode and keep the energy flowing. In addition, it calms your brain, enhances digestive function, build up the shoulders, shape your abs, and stretches your spine and neck.

Forward Bending Pose (Uttanasana)

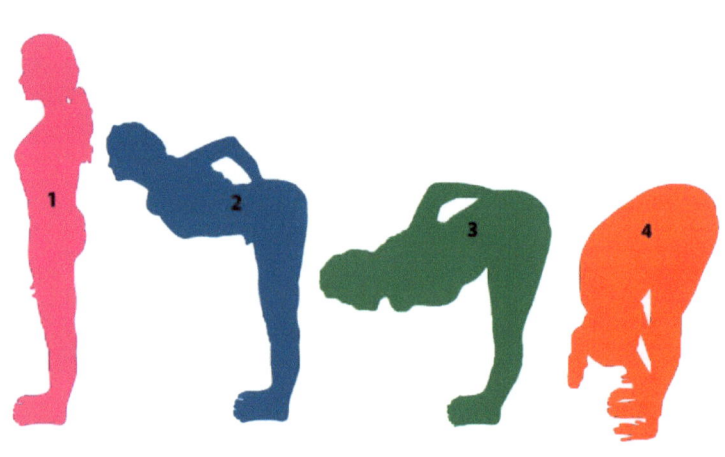

Avoid: You would be well-advised to stay away from this particular pose if you have any sort of abdomen illness, neck injury or high blood pressure.

In step 1, get started by standing on the ground straightly, where your big toes should be touched together, spread your toes, and use a little gap in between your heels. Balance your upper part of the body over your pelvis and maintain straightforward alignment.

In step 2-3, bring your hands to your hips, take a deep breath, exhale and bend forward from the hips. As you move towards the ground draw front torso out of the hips and open the space between the pubis and the top of the sternum.

In step 4, when you are completely folded over your legs, bring your palms and fingertips towards the ground beside your feet. This won't be very easy to do; however, if you continue trying to do it then progressively you will be able to achieve this performance posture. Continue pressing your heels firmly into the ground, buttocks towards the ceiling, holding this posture and taking deep breaths. Move your head, shoulder and chest a little up when you are breathing in. When you are exhaling, continue bending to the knees, where your forehead should touch your knees, and hold this posture for about 10-20 seconds. Don't keep you head down for more than 40-60 seconds because it rushes blood to your head. When you are done, lift your hands on your waist, inhale and gradually go back to your standing position (step 1) again.

Benefits: This is a valuable exercise to shape your abdomen muscles. It can help you relax by flowing blood into your head.

Warrior Pose (Virabhadrasana)

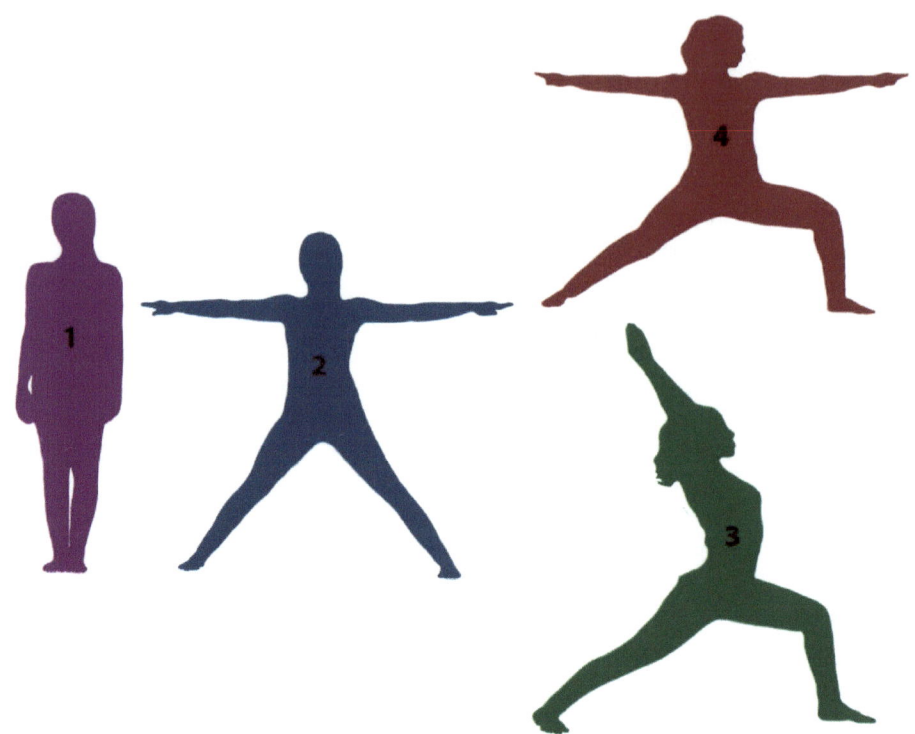

Avoid: You would be well-advised to stay away from this particular pose if you have any sort of leg, knee, and back injury.

Warrior Pose (A)

In step 1-2, get started by standing straightly and then moving one of your leg sideways apart from your other leg where your legs should be parallel to each other. Afterward, gradually lift your both hands up where your arms should be parallel to the ground.

In step 3, turn your left foot laterally and slowly twist your hips and torso towards left along with your both hands by maintaining the posture of your hands.

Now slowly bend your left knee and move your hips and upper body in that direction. Your right thigh should be parallel and look on your left side. Take a few breaths in this posture and then raise your both hands towards the ceiling. Your palms should be attached with one another and take a few breaths again.

When you are done, return to your standing position by gently reversing the process. Relax and do the steps (1, 2 and 3) by bending your right knee this time.

Warrior Pose (B)

In step 1-2, get started by standing straightly and then moving one of your leg sideways apart from your other leg where your legs should be parallel to each other. Afterward, gradually lift your both hands up where your arms should be parallel to the ground.

In step 4, turn your left foot laterally, slowly bend you left knee and move your hips and upper body in that direction by maintaining the posture of your hands. This time doesn't twist your hips and upper body. You may look on your left. Maintain 90-degree angle within your left foot whereas you right foot should be parallel on the ground (like a slope) and continue having a few breaths. When you are done, slowly come back to your first standing position and continue steps (1, 2, and 4) again on the right side.

Benefits: This particular exercise is a good one to strengthen your knees. It also stretches your arms, shoulders, thighs and abdomen.

Plough Pose (Halasana)

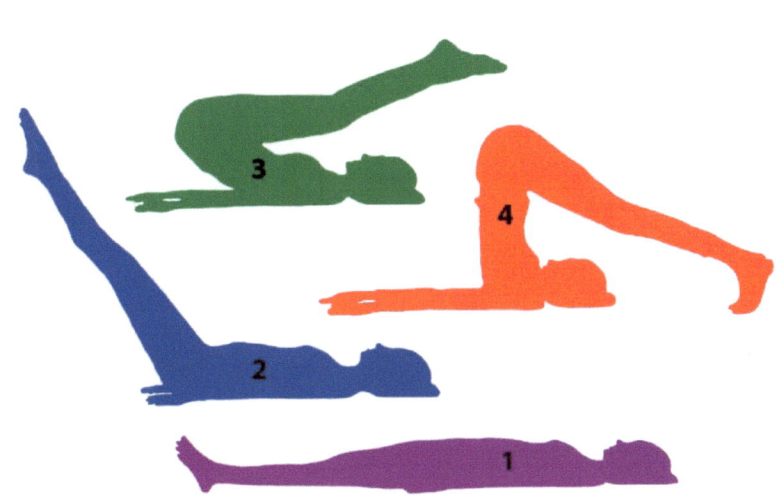

Avoid: You would be well-advised to stay away from this particular pose if you have any sort of head, neck injury, hypertension, and liver disorders.

Step 1 - Get started by lying down on your back in a straight line. Bring your legs together, feet should be touched together, and hands close to your body pressed down on the ground.

In step 2-4, keep your head, shoulder and arms pressed down on the ground, exhale, gradually raise your feet towards the ceiling without bending your knees, take your feet towards the back of your head and touch the ground using your toes. Maintain you buttocks towards the ceiling in a straightforward way by completely balancing your weight on your shoulder and hands. You will find yourself in a plow shape here. Hold your position for about 30 seconds and gently return back to your lying position again when you are done.

Benefits: This pose tones the muscles of your buttock and strengthens your shoulders and thighs. It also stimulates the functioning of the thyroid glands, parathyroid glands, lungs and abdominal organs, therefore helping the blood rush to your head and face, improves digestion and keeps the hormonal levels in check.

Sun Salutation (Surya namaskar)

Avoid: You would be well-advised to stay away from this particular pose if you have any sort of injury related to previous yoga poses.

This exercise is actually a combination of the above-mentioned exercises which are performed in sequence.

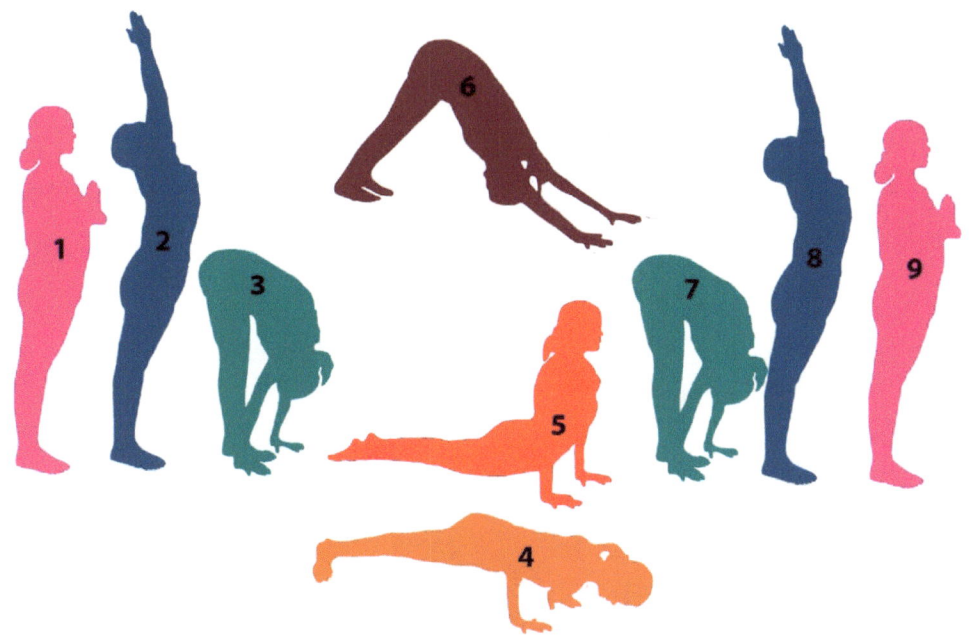

Surya namaskar or sun salutation (A)

Step 1 - Stand straightly on the ground, keep your feet together, and palms in front of your chest just like namaskar.

Step 2 - Breathe in, raise both of your arms above your head towards the ceiling, press the palms together, look up, and try stretching to go a little higher.

In step 3, breathe out and go down to forward bending pose by keeping your both palms next to your feet (Please, check the details in the Forward Bending Pose).

Step 4 - From forward bending pose, bend both knees, look onward and jump back to downward dog posture and then to low push-up posture where your legs, hips, backbone, neck and head should be straight by pressing on your both palms.

In step 5, breathe in, look ahead and gently raise your head and shoulder towards the ceiling. Your legs and hips should go down; however, they should not touch the ground and try lifting your thighs up. Hold this position for about 20-30 seconds.

In step 6, breathe out, return back to downward dog position by grounding your heels a little closer, push your palms away from you, lock your chin towards your chest, and take a few breaths by holding this position.

Step 7 - Now bend both knees towards your hips, look forward and jump back to forward bending position. Step 8 and 9 - Breathe in, lift your head and torso upwards to a standing position again.

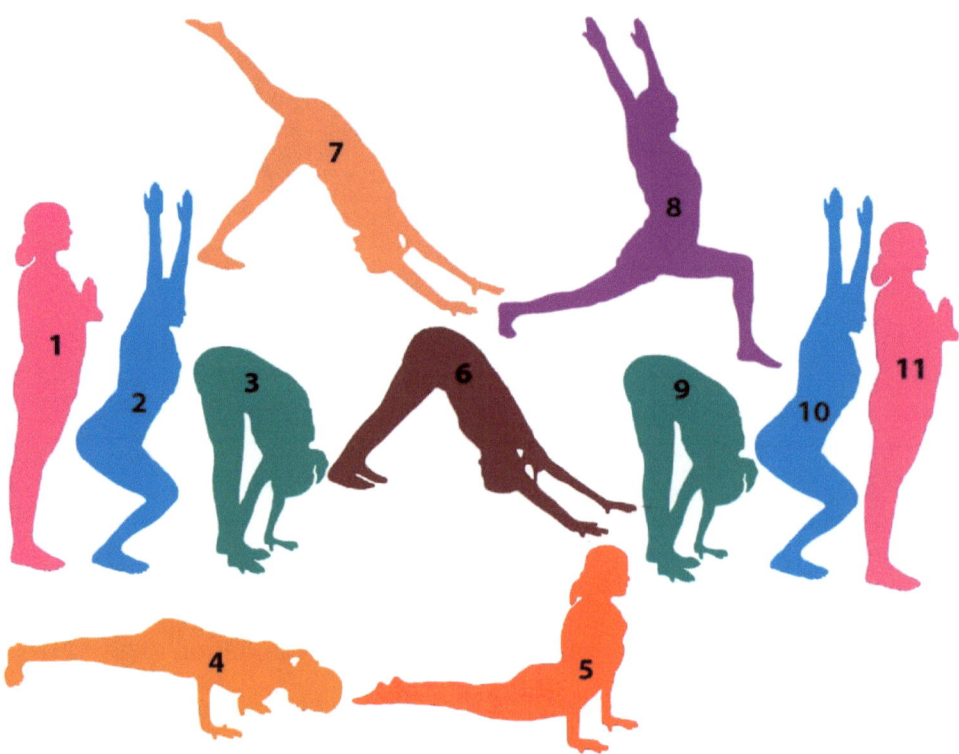

Surya namaskar or sun salutation (B)

Step 1 - Stand straightly on the ground, keep your feet together, big toes should be touched side by side, palms in front of your chest.

In step 2, inhale, raise both of your arms above your head towards the ceiling, bend your knees, buttocks pushed back, fingers are stretched towards the ceiling, maintain gaps in between your hands, and try to perform the chair yoga pose (Please, check the details in the Chair Pose).

Step 3 - Breathe out and go down to forward bending pose by keeping your both palms next to your feet (Please, check the details in the [Forward Bending Pose](#)).

Step 4 - From forward bending pose, bend both knees, look forward and jump back to downward dog posture and then to low push-up posture where your legs, hips, backbone, neck and head should be straight by pressing on your both palms.

Step 5 - Breathe in, look forward and slowly raise your head and shoulder towards the ceiling. Your legs and hips should go down; however, they should not touch the ground and try lifting your thighs up. Hold this posture for about 20-30 seconds.

Step 6 - Breathe out, return back to downward dog posture by grounding your heels a little closer, push your palms away from you, lock your chin towards your chest, and take a few breaths by holding this posture.

Step 7 - From this posture, you can raise your right leg up and hold for about 10-20 seconds.

Step 8 - Now take a big step forward by using the same leg which was lifted earlier, look forward, breathe in, lift your head, shoulder and both hands like the chair pose. Take a few breaths here and return to downward dog posture. From here you can repeat the last two steps for your left leg.

Step 9 - Now bend both knees towards your hips from downward dog posture, look forward and jump back to forward bending posture.

Step 10 - Breathe in, lift your head and torso upwards back to chair pose again.

Step 11 - Afterward return to standing position.

You are welcome to perform three to five of these above-mentioned yoga steps from sun salutation (a) or (b) in a regular basis.

Action Plan

According to estimates, if your weight is 200 pounds and you continue performing regular yoga workouts for an hour then you will approximately burn 150-250 kcal including BMR. Even though yoga or power yoga is a slow process of shedding pounds quickly compared to cardiovascular workouts, many practitioners strongly believe yoga can help people to lose weight.

It requires around 15 hours of yoga exercises to lose just 1 pound or 0.45 kg of body weight. As a result, it would be a wise choice to mix other workouts along with yoga exercises to lose a significant amount of weight at a good pace.

How to start yoga exercises as a beginner?

Yoga related tips:
- For a breath of fresh air, the better choice is to do it in an open space where you can breathe in (inhale) deeply and breathe out (exhale) slowly.
- Don't ever forget to relax as soon as you are feeling exhausted or fatigued.
- Constantly try to look for your breaking points, different holding positions during yoga where your body is being challenged; however, not stressed. Maintain an open mindset as soon as you figure this out.
- Discover how to have the deep feelings of motion while performing even the smallest movements.
- Exercise within an area with no mirrors, and focus on the inner experience instead of external routine performance.
- Realize that you are not only doing this for losing weight but also for improving abilities such as stamina, self-control, compassion, meditation, and so on.
- It is better to fix specific dates and time within a week for only yoga workout and follow that schedule.

Chapter 07: Swimming to lose weight

It is in no way very late to master or enhance your swimming abilities. Swimming to lose weight is definitely possible, a soothing form of exercise, and full of excitement. Swimming is really a powerful exercise because it combines exercising nearly, on the whole, body such as heart, lungs, and entire body muscles. Exercising in water involves your cardiovascular system and muscles to function in a separate way compared to exercising on land. Swimming necessitates entire body muscles within your body to operate together in order to help keep you moving, breathing and staying afloat. You will be able to burn an extra amount of calories because after swimming your body is going to use more energy to recover your muscle tissues.

Swimming does not work sometimes. Why?
1) Swimmers tend to feel very hungry after swimming and they continue to consume a lot of extra calories besides their daily intake of calories. Swimming to lose weight won't work if you continue to consume more calories.
2) Swimmers tend to feel exhausted after swimming and they don't intend to carry on their other physical workouts to lose weight.

Health benefits of swimming

- Swimming is a first-rate muscular and cardiovascular workout for your cardiovascular system
- Regular swimmers look younger than their actual age
- It reduces the risk of type 2 diabetes, heart diseases and stroke.
- Swimming is relaxing and less injurious compared to other workouts or strength workouts

Swimming Set

- Swimsuit: get a nice and comfortable swimsuit
- Goggles: to increase your underwater eyesight and protect your eyes from chlorine water
- Cap: necessary to swim, breathe smoothly and to protect your hair
- Ear plugs: necessary if you are vulnerable to ear infections
- Water bottle: Water adds no calories at all. So, maintain your body hydrated by drinking enough water.

Safety for beginners

- Don't try to swim alone to learn swimming
- Don't swim in the swimming pool where it is out of your own depth
- Don't attempt to race with other swimmers and have respect for all other swimmers around you
- Don't try to learn swimming in open water, rivers, or lakes

Action Plan

If your weight is 200 pounds then you will be able to burn approximately 400-700 calories per hour in a 25 degrees Celsius swimming pool by normal freestyle swimming and including BMR. It depends on your overall body weight, swimming strokes such as freestyle, breaststroke, backstroke, mixed strokes, swimming speed and temperature of water. Swimming in cold water burns 20%-30% more calories. But you need to prepare yourself to stay out of hypothermia.

Look for your nearest local swimming pool and choose your suitable group, dates, and time. If you are absolutely new to swimming then talk to the swimming instructor of that pool or you can request one of your family members or relatives who can teach you how to swim. Gather three required items namely swimsuit, goggles, and cap in order to get started from the next available schedule. Mastering the abilities of different swimming strokes is really fascinating. It might become a lot more interesting if you have a swimming partner whose focus is swimming to lose weight as well.

An important fact for a successful swim schedule is actually splitting regular swim time into smaller sections where you should mix verities of swimming strokes, speed and rest time periods.

You know how to calculate your daily intake of calories. So, create your own desirable and flexible swimming schedules, for example, half an hour on 3-5 specific days within a week to lose weight besides other physical workouts.

Chapter 08: Cycling to lose weight

If you have a childhood passion where you and your friends used to spend whole days tearing up the roads then you can naturally prefer cycling to lose weight. It is not really hard to ride bicycle or mountain bike every now and then besides walking, running and swimming. Cycling will make you exhausted and your legs will hurt including your butt; however, it will help you to lose weight.

It might seem to you, riding a bike is a relatively slow process of losing weight. But it is an effective one when you mix it along with your other exercises to lose weight. Because there are people who really lost 100 to 100+ pounds just by riding a bicycle and keeping simple diet plan.

By following rudimentary rules of nutrition to remain healthy to keep riding strong, you would acquire the most out of your cycling, and to lose weight in the procedure.

Health benefits of cycling

- Cycling is an outstanding cardiovascular workout for leg muscle growth, increased fitness, and staying slim.
- Cycling is environmentally friendly compared to other automobiles.
- It can save your regular expenses on transportation or purchasing fuel.
- It helps to reduce sleeplessness, hypertension, and others.

Action Plan

According to general estimates, if your weight is 200 pounds and you continue cycling for an hour at 6 miles/hour or 9.6 km/hour then you will approximately burn 300-400 calories including BMR.

After 6 hours of cycling in a week, you will be able to burn 1800-2400 kcal because it depends on riding hours, riding speed, distance covered, and body weight. It takes 3500-3600 kcal in order to shed 1 pound. So, you will be able to shed half a pound or 0.45 kg in a week just after cycling for 6 hours. Use the optional tips from running to lose weight.

You can purchase a bicycle and related clothing which fits & ensures your comfort. You are welcome to consult with a local bicycle expert before purchasing a well-fitting bicycle and clothing. Bicycles can be of various types such as:

- Road bike or Racing bike: price ranges from $300 to $1500+
- Mountain bike: $500+
- Folding bike: $800+
- Touring bike: $800 to $2000+
- Hybrid bike: $200 to $1500+
- Cargo bike: $1000+
- others

For safety precautions, you need to know bicycle friendly routes in your local area by getting bike maps from the bike shops or from Google Maps.

You can try to ride bicycle or mountain bike for at least 60 minutes with different intensity levels.

Adopt a "better than zero" mindset. Say you set out for 9 miles. "If you get tired after 6, you can stop—but 6 is still better than zero.

Your ride would be more comfortable, natural and it would go by fast if you pick a great scenery area, listen to news or music, and have someone to join with you.

There should be typical beginner challenges, like sitting on the narrower saddle, stopping, putting your foot down, and bicycle maintenance.

Don't forget to use your log book wisely to note the date, time, cycling hours, and distance covered. Afterward find out the intensity of cycling and calories burned by cycling.

Useful Tips

- A better approach is to have your nutritious and healthy meal before you ride because you won't have the required fuel if you miss it and exercise is supposed to speed up your metabolism.
- Instead of continuing without snacks, chocolate, beverage or else, you can limit your portions to consume them.
- Always secure your bicycle in a parking area with multi-locks and if possible then keep it indoors.
- Learn the basics of bicycle maintenance such as breakdowns, chain maintenance, and tire inflation as early as possible to deal with those in a regular basis.
- Use bicycle related clothing to stay away from discomfort and chafe rash.

Chapter 09: Weekly Calculation

Weekly Chart	Regular Physical Exercises that includes (kcal) *[This is an example chart]*										Other Physical Activities (kcal)	Daily Intake of Calories (kcal)		Result (Daily) Kcal [Considering BMR is 1900 kcal]
	Walking		Running		Yoga		Swimming		Cycling					
Week Days	Time (M/E), Length (L), Distance Covered (DC)	Done (Y/N), Calories Burned (CB)	Time (M/E), Length (L), Distance Covered (DC)	Done (Y/N), Calories Burned (CB)	Time, Yoga Pose Name (YPN), Length (L)	Done (Y/N), Calories Burned (CB)	Time (M/E), Length (L), Distance Covered (DC)	Done (Y/N), Calories Burned (CB)	Time (M/E), Length (L), Distance Covered (DC)	Done (Y/N), Calories Burned (CB)	Don't forget to include all other physical activities (Playing, Driving, Dancing and so on)	Breakfast(B), Lunch(L), Dinner(D), Snacks(S), Others including drinks(O)	Total intake (TIC) (kcal)	Total intake of calories (TIC) – Total expenditure of calories (BMR + TEF + Physical Exercises)
Saturday		N		N	E, All Poses, L-30 min	Y, 100	M, L-30 min, DC-600 m	Y, CB-300		N	200	B – 600 kcal, L – 700, D – 500, S – 100, O - 300	2200	TIC-2200 –[BMR-1900 + TEF-200 + PE-600] = - 500
Sunday		N		N	E, All Poses, L-30 min	Y, 100	M, L-30 min, DC-600 m	Y, CB-300		N	200	B – 600 kcal, L – 600, D – 500, S – 200, O - 300	2200	TIC-2200 –[BMR-1900 + TEF-200 + PE-600] = - 500
Monday	M, L-30 min, DC-2.5 km	Y, CB-150	M, L-30 min, DC-5 km	Y, CB-300		N		N	E, L-30 min, DC-5 km	Y, CB-200	200	B – 700 kcal, L – 700, D – 500, S – 200, O - 200	2300	TIC-2300 –[BMR-1900 + TEF-200 + PE-850] = - 650
Tuesday		N		N	E, All Poses, L-30 min	Y, 100	M, L-30 min, DC-600 m	Y, CB-300		N	200	B – 700 kcal, L – 600, D – 500, S – 100, O - 200	2100	TIC-2100 –[BMR-1900 + TEF-200 + PE-600] = - 600
Wednesday	M, L-30 min, DC-2.5 km	Y, CB-150	M, L-30 min, DC-5 km	Y, CB-300		N		N	E, L-30 min, DC-5 km	Y, CB-200	200	B – 700 kcal, L – 700, D – 500, S – 200, O - 200	2300	TIC-2300 –[BMR-1900 + TEF-200 + PE-850] = - 650
Thursday		N		N	E, All Poses, L-30 min	Y, 100	M, L-30 min, DC-600 m	Y, CB-300		N	200	B – 700 kcal, L – 700, D – 500, S – 100, O - 200	2200	TIC-2200 –[BMR-1900 + TEF-200 + PE-600] = - 500
Friday	M, L-30 min, DC-2.5 km	Y, CB-150	M, L-30 min, DC-5 km	Y, CB-300		N		N	E, L-30 min, DC-5 km	Y, CB-200	200	B – 700 kcal, L – 600, D – 500, S – 300, O - 200	2300	TIC-2300 –[BMR-1900 + TEF-200 + PE-850] = - 650

The above-mentioned table is an example of your weekly calculation. Your calculations should be similar like this; however, the intention of this person (whose body weight - 200 pounds, age - 30 years, body height – 6 feet 2 inch, BMR – 1900 kcal daily when completely resting) is to lose 1 pound in each week. His desire is to lose 20 pounds in 20 weeks or by 5 months. This is a very standard process of losing a significant amount of weight comfortably and without causing any illness or injury. You can also include the temperature of water of the swimming pool to track down everything more specifically.

What should be your weekly aim to lose weight?

1) You must have a good plan first because you don't want to trouble your existing everyday life or work.
2) No matter what you must not gain additional weight just by overeating
3) No matter what you must not starve in order to lose weight quickly

4) No matter what you must not hurt yourself, cause illness, stress or injury to lose weight

5) Your well-being is the first priority and then losing weight at a standard pace like 1 pound in each week.

6) Have a thorough conversation with your doctor first before working on your unique and customized weekly plan because you might have existing health issues or hidden health facts where it should be dealt with precautions and proper care.

7) Try to lose only half pound in your very first week and make sure you are being fantastic after those hours of workout. Focus on losing 1 pound from the second week, check your health status in a regular basis and be consistent with this target until you are done with losing your expected pounds.

8) Don't hesitate to visit your doctor if you feel any pain, discomfort, stress, and fatigue at any point which requires doctors' attention.

9) Stay away from any particular exercise if you don't enjoy it, or it is causing trouble for you. You can do the adjustment by decreasing your total intake of calories and increasing other daily workout hours slightly.

10) You need to have a strong determination and focus on losing weight and controlling intake of calories.

11) A better way is not to cut off food that you love and instead just reduce the quantity and rate.

12) The smart approach is to split your regular workout hours instead of only morning or evening or etc. The study shows that splitting hours twice is better and effective compared to daily workouts for a long time.

13) Get a friend or friends, he or she can be family members, relatives, co-workers, neighbors who also wants to lose weight, follow the things that motivate you, add other things that interest you in order to have fun and pass your entire workout hours with full of life.

How do you calculate further from this table?

You already know that you have to burn 3500 - 3600 kcal to shed 1 pound. So, if you can manage to burn 500 kcal in a regular basis then you are supposed to burn 3500 kcal in 7 days.

According to the table, that person is supposed to burn 500 + 500 + 650 + 600 + 650 + 500 + 650 = 4050 kcal in one week. However, you have to refine the calculation more because in each exercise hour the BMR was included. His BMR is 1900 kcal and it is based on 24 hours. So, his BMR in each hour is supposed to be 1900 kcal / 24 hours = 80 kcal / hour. He must have exercised for 8.5 hours within that week.

He was very careful and calculative regarding daily intake of calories. He exercised for 8.5 hours and managed to burn the following amount of calories in a week:

= [4050 – (80 x 8.5)] kcal
= (4050 – 680) kcal
= 3370 kcal

Therefore, he is looking forward to shedding 1 pound after each week by having balanced micronutrients, calorie-controlled diet plan, and doing cardio exercises such as walking, running, yoga, swimming, and cycling. He didn't do a lot of other physical activities, which are directly related to the expenditure of calories, on each day. That is why, his other physical activities burned average 200 kcal. **You must not miss to include other physical activities (playing, driving, dancing, strength workouts, talking, etc.) in your grand calculation.** These other physical activities can be discussed in the future books as well.

What do you have to do if you want to shed more than 1 pound in each week?

You might be tempted to do so. But it is strongly recommended that you try to lose just 1 pound in each week. If you insist on doing so then you can do the followings:

1) You must talk to your doctor regarding the type of exercises, your diet plan, your desires to lose weight in a short period of time, and make sure you will stay healthy and don't cause unnecessary injury in your journey.
2) Reduce your daily intake of calories by having fewer snacks and beverages. Never reduce too much from your three important meals of the day, especially not from the breakfast. But be careful to maintain your balanced micronutrients. Make sure you are determined to burn calories only to lose unnecessary weight and water weight instead of losing muscle tissues.
3) Increase your physical workout hours gradually based on your stamina. But watch out for any unnecessary injury, fatigue, stress, or any sort of problem. Take extra care when you are performing intensive workouts including strength workouts.
4) Things might go south if you burn more than 800 kcal or take 800 kcal less than your daily caloric requirement (BMR + TEF + Physical Exercises) because each person is unique and his or her body metabolism might not support the imbalance of calories. Please, talk to your doctor first about this and plan your further

activities.

What do you have to do after shedding your desired pounds?

It is totally up to you and feel free to maintain your healthy and happy lifestyle. Or, you can do the followings in relation to controlling calories:

1) You can continue your exercises if you enjoy it. Just make sure your daily intake of calories is equal and not going to be higher than the daily expenditure of calories.
2) Or, you can reduce your exercises and make sure you are going to burn equal calories or 50-100 kcal more.
3) Or, you can change your exercises to give yourself a handsome or gorgeous look.

Conclusion

Thanks for downloading the book and reading it!

I hope this book "Weight Loss Smart Workbook - How to lose weight by eating low carbs, calorie-controlled diet plan, exercises – walking, running, swimming, yoga & cycling" was able to help you to learn how to lose weight by eating low carbs, low fat, calculating calories in diet plan, and cardio exercises.

Once again, three simple key points:
1) Somehow control your daily intake of calories.
2) Consume balanced micronutrients that you enjoy.
3) Continue physical exercises in a regular basis that you enjoy.

Remember, you have a choice to stick to your weight loss plan.

You will be making relatively good progress if you can stay away from foods that are not suitable to lose weight, follow a calorie-controlled diet plan, and do your regular physical exercises.

Technically, you have to stand for yourself. No one can help you until you don't help yourself. Believe in yourself and do what is best for you to make progress. Believe in math, small progress at a time will be counted as a big progress and might give a healthy and happy life for you and people around you. Increase strength to love you and others for real.

If you enjoyed this book and found it useful, then I would like to ask you for a quick favor.

Would you be kind enough to spare a little time and post a short review on Amazon?

In fact, all reviews are important for future publications & editions where your opinion & support matters. I personally read each review. I would like to see your valuable review and suggestions.

Please, take a moment and be sure to post a review as feedback so that I can make this and future books even better.

A better approach is to split a long term goal into specific small goals in order to track down your overall progress or results. **Don't forget to reward yourself after shedding 5 pounds or 2.25 kg each time**. Smile honestly for your own hard work and continue losing weight like that in order to live an awesome and healthy lifestyle.

Congratulations! You have finished reading the book! **Lose weight & have a healthy lifestyle!**

Sincere thanks and good luck!

www.ingramcontent.com/pod-product-compliance
Lightning Source LLC
Chambersburg PA
CBHW050817290526
45792CB00001B/157